# Foreword

"Research", a word that is both fascinating and daunting. Fascinating because it suggests delving into deep mysteries and the dreams of becoming famous. Daunting because it's like an ocean, one does not readily know where to begin, which direction to sail and which ports to call upon. I began my research career as a graduate student trying to come up with a blood test to detect pancreatic cancer. Although I was not entirely successful in achieving that goal, it took me on a journey that introduced me to different kinds of people, to different tools of research, to the dark depths of failure and the exhilarating heights of discovery. It helped me turn my passion of writing into something useful. It helped satisfy my curiosity to find answers to my questions about health. It became a part of my life and ultimately my passion. When I started residency, I was not sure how I would ever find time to carry on this passion. But I did, and today, nearly fifty published articles and a book chapter later, I would like to share my story. I hope others will benefit from it, and not be daunted by the term "research". I think we should call it "discovery" but then again, that's just me......

# Table of contents

1. Foreword
2. Beginnings
3. Why should I do research?
4. Where should I start?
5. Personal tips for success in Research
   a) Choose something to research/write about that you are passionately interested in
   b) Be organized
   c) Plan your research in chunks
   d) Use whatever research time you have to do something, however small the task
   e) Make a start
   f) Set deadlines
   g) Work on your abstract
   h) Include informative schematics and learn the art of drawing "electronically
   i) Choose a mentor
   j) Attend conferences
   k) Take courses related to your area of interest
6. Preparing your first poster- a case report
7. Preparing your first manuscript
8. Funding
9. Sample Cover letter
10. Conclusion
11. About the author

# Beginning...

In my third year of medical school, we learnt about pathology. The science that deals with the microscopic and macroscopic features of disease and with the mechanisms driving disease occurrence fascinated me. I remember one of the first chapters in our textbook was on cell death, a process called apoptosis. I remember looking at the beautiful schematic diagram of a cell undergoing the various stages of regulated cell death, and thinking "what do the terms tumor suppressor, oncogene, and p53 mean?" I was intrigued and no matter how many times I read it I could not really understand what was going on inside the cells. I liked the gross pathology and looking at slides of diseased tissues stained with various dyes. But somehow I felt a part of my understanding was missing- the part that dealt with understanding the pathways that drove these disease processes, or "molecular pathology".

Emptiness followed me through the rest of medical school. I always felt that if only I could grasp how things work at the level of a cell I could understand many of the disease processes better. When I was done with my bachelors in medicine, I had an opportunity to decide what I wanted to do next. Quite serendipitously, I received an invitation for pursuing a graduate program in Biochemistry and Molecular Biology from Nebraska. Little did I know that I was embarking on an odyssey.

I spent six years in the graduate program working on various aspects of applied research. Then, I started my residency program at the Nebraska Medical Center. During the three years of my training, I felt a need among my fellow residents of a guide to research, not a cookbook but rather a guide that would be helpful even to a novice. I hope to share my experiences in this book and provide residents and other aspiring young researchers with my perspective about how to begin research. Like everything, one improves with repetition and I hope that the readers will use this book as a guide to launch a fun filled journey into the unknown....

# Basic questions

Having gone from a phase where I did not know anything about biomedical research to one where it has become a hobby for me, I would ask someone who is thinking of foraying into the area of research ask themselves a question- why are you getting into this? I think it's a fundamental question. In whatever activity you commit yourself to in your life, there needs to be a purpose. The key thing about research is that it's nearly always an all or none thing. Some people immerse themselves in it and work tirelessly their entire life searching for answers. Some do it temporarily as a means to an end and then realize it is not really their cup of tea. My reason for doing it- I was very interested in the word "research". That's how I started. I just knew that I wanted to know how research is done. I read the well known textbooks of medicine and at the end of each chapter there was the section of references. I would read those and wonder about the great people who wrote those works of science that today we are reading! In school, we read about great Indian scientists, Dr C.V. Raman and Dr. Jagadish Chandra Bose, about stalwarts like Einstein and Bohr and later on came to know about people like Stephen Hawkins and Edwin Hubble. As you can see, only one among them was a biologist, that too a botanist. Nonetheless, the wonder of discovery was what drew me in. I was not even sure if I would last because in my opinion, researchers are the cream of society. Their discoveries are what drive mankind from one era to another. After entering into the field of scientific research, I had a chance to make another choice, this time as I was getting ready to enter residency in Internal Medicine- do I become a clinician and let my skills and knowledge gained through work in the laboratory just be a thing of the past or do I try to apply what I had learnt on the bench in the clinical scenario and try a marriage of the two? I have chosen the latter. And when I asked myself the quintessential question- "Why did I make that choice?" the answer was clear to me, it was because I enjoyed research and I enjoy writing. So scientific research and scientific writing is my hobby. I urge you, the reader to also think prospectively as to why you want to do what you want to do. Once you have that clear, the fog will lift and you will find it's not really a struggle, you just needed a clear perspective. In the following sections, I will try to answer some questions first, and then move on to personal tips for success in research and in scientific writing.

# Why should I do research?

I think that is an important question one needs to ask themselves. Each one has a different reason- some do it so that they can distinguish their application as they apply for fellowship. Some do it to stand out in the eyes of their peers and program leadership. Some because they like working with a particular physician whom they see as their mentor. Still others do it because they love asking questions and finding answers.

When I came to the United States for the first time, I came with a goal of learning more about what happens at the molecular level in a cell. I was interested to know what research was having not really had any exposure to biomedical journals during my schooling. All I knew was that I wanted to learn something new and do "research". I did not know at that time that I would fall in love with it. Over the years I have posed the question "Why do you do research?" to numerous colleagues and friends. I found that nearly all my graduate school colleagues answered that they simply liked the intrigue of discovery. My resident friends usually reported that their interest was driven by an interest in a competitive fellowship. As I alluded to before, have a clear idea of what your goals are. Some people like to write things down, while others think through in their head. Either way, think of the long term implications- are you willing to devote a certain fraction of your time (typically, 1-2 full days in one month) for research during your residency? Or do you want to do something to complete an academic requirement and then be done with it? Either way, the book will be helpful to you. The purpose here is not to selectively encourage those who want to devote a career towards research. Rather, my goal is to have a discussion with you, the reader and share some experiences, some things that I learnt from my experiences with you and help you flow into research rather than make a jarring landing.

# Where should I start?

That is one of the fundamental questions that came to my mind as I began wetting my feet in the field of research. I remember meeting different professors during my research rotations at the university. Each one of them spoke about their research and gave me articles to read. Although I could not tell them on their face, the truth was that I could not understand any of the technical things they spoke about. But I did not want to look like an idiot of course! So, I took those articles and went home and read them. I found them exceedingly difficult and boring. At every step, there was a word I could not understand. After some time, I just gave up trying. Often I would fall asleep reading the articles. Knowing myself, I knew that it was because these articles were not igniting a fire inside me. The reason- because they were written in such technical jargon that I could not understand, and what I could not understand, I could not like or enjoy. That taught me my first valuable lesson of research- whenever you do something is ready to explain it in very simple terms to a layman.

Coming back to our question- I started with rotating through every lab. While I am sure the lab was looking to get me interested in their research, what I was seeking out was a mentor- someone who would understand that I was a blank slate and would teach me from the basics; not just the how's but the why's. In most labs where I worked, I came across teachers who were too busy in their work to teach me the whys. I was given a manual, taught a technique and asked to repeat it. I felt that I was just someone helping them with a technique. Again, this left me disinterested as it was not fulfilling my deepest desire at that time, for a mentor. Just when I had almost given up, I began work in Dr Batra's lab. I was immediately struck by Dr Batra's quality of explaining his research in simple terms to me. That immediately excited me; I wanted to do something too! But, being a novice I felt helpless. That's when Dr Batra assigned me to Christopher Nemos. He was a post doctoral fellow in the lab and at that time was working on peripheral blood mononuclear cells isolated from patients who were either healthy or had pancreatic cancer. Using a technique called Real time PCR which he had perfected, he was looking for expression of a particular gene (these are portions of the DNA that code for proteins which in turn are the building blocks of life) in the blood cells of healthy individuals and those with pancreatic cancer. The hypothesis was that if the level of this gene was higher in cancer patients, we could potentially use it as a blood test to detect early stage pancreatic cancer. It seemed so clinically relevant, I was hooked. During the month that I spent in the lab, I worked hard. And it was not glamorous, mostly pipetting water from a reservoir into a plastic plate that had 96 tiny wells. I used to do that again and again. The goal was to be good at pipetting because the test itself relied on accuracy of volume. The volume was in microliters, smaller than a drop of water and my Chris told me that he needed to be confident that I was going to be accurate in pipetting before he would let me near the patient samples.

From this experience, I learnt that when you do not know where to start, one option is to take time to explore available options. Some of them may not make sense to you; some of the topics not interest you. But ultimately, it may just be the personality of the person you work with that draws you towards a research project. Some people, like me are not too critical and instead ready to accept failures as easily as success. This has helped me in every phase of life both professional and personal. But that's a story for another day.

# Personal tips for success in research

# Tip 1. Choose something to research/write about that you are passionately interested in

For instance, I am really interested in understanding the relationship between biochemical tests used to assess liver function and abnormalities in blood counts. The reason is that I see a lot of patients with abnormal liver function tests (LFTs) that also seem to have some abnormalities in their red, white blood cell or platelet count. Once I knew what I wanted to research on, the next step was laying out what all I needed to answer my research.

| Question | Solution |
|---|---|
| Where will I find sufficient number of patients who have information about blood cell counts and liver function tests? | Searched the internet and found that the National Health and Nutrition Examination Survey (NHANES) study conducted by the CDC maintains this kind of information and best of all it is free for public use! |
| Where will I find instructions on how to access the data from the database | NHANES has very helpful instructions on how to open data files and interpret study codes |
| How do I find which software to use | Mostly something of a trial and error or based on one's familiarity. I mostly use SPSS and the student version works just great. |
| How do I know what kind of tests to use? | Read up on studies that have examined similar questions, for instance "relationship between exercise duration and BMI" and see what kind of tests they employed. Also helpful to read up on internet blogs and of course help option included with the statistical software |

I have included an example where I used an online database. But you could do research using patient databases available in your hospital. In most cases that involve human subjects you have to get approval from your institutional review board (IRB). But you can also do research that does not require IRB approval. For instance, you could investigate "the role of online forums in internal medicine residency interview planning" wherein you would observe data available on internet forums to investigate for instance, what the most important areas that interview candidates focus on in their discussion. You could also write a review article on your area of interest. We will cover how to plan on writing a particular kind of article in another section.

# Tip 2. Be organized

In today's fast paced world, we are constantly shifting focus from one area to another. For instance, a resident may have to focus on his inpatients in the morning, then on notes, then on a conference topic, then on his clinic patients, then again on notes and then on his family. In the midst of all this, if one has to focus on research, it could become a daunting task especially since a large part of being a researcher is knowing how to organize your work and how to prioritize. For instance, in the beginning of my research career, I found it hard to do anything productive because most of my time was spent in reading up on articles. It was hard because I felt I was not doing anything. For some people, that may be hard. But it's a necessary part of being a researcher. You have to give time to learning certain skills. Then, like in any other trade, you practice them, again and again. Once you are good at the basics, then you begin applying these individual skills to create a complete research project. For instance, let's take the previous example of my project "investigating the relationship between variations in liver function tests and occurrence of low red cell, white cell or platelet counts". I could divide the study components into

- Data collection
- Data analysis (biostatistics) and interpretation
- Background information
- Manuscript preparation
- References
- Preparing to submit for peer review

At each step, it's important to be organized.

1. **Data collection:**
   The NHANES database (used for the study mentioned above) has files divided year wise. For instance, 1999-2000, 2001-2002 and so on. For each year, there are separate files for liver function tests, blood counts and demographics (i.e. age, race, gender and the like). You have to organize your area of storage- typically the hard drive of your computer or an external drive into individual folders with easily identifiable names (e.g. "1999" is the main folder with sub folder "liver

tests"). Needless to say, make sure your area of storage is dependable and for data containing patient identifiers, make sure they are stored on encrypted disks. Drives do crash and I suggest you make copies of your data from time to time on DVDs or another storage device.

2. **Data analysis (biostatistics) and interpretation**
Once you have all the data, you need to organize it before starting any analysis. For me, I first consolidate files in a given year (e.g. "liver tests", "blood counts" from 1999) into a single file. Next, consolidate files from multiple years into a single file (e.g. from 1999-2010). Then, exclude duplicate cases. Next, make a list of tests to run on the data. This is helpful as many times you will need to convert continuous data (e.g. age, weight, blood pressure) into categorical data (e.g. body mass index, low normal or high blood pressure). I always maintain a notepad document in which I write down the name of the original variable (e.g. weight), the variable I coded it into (e.g. BMI) and the categories I created (e.g. BMI between 18-24: normal, 24.1-29.9: overweight and ≥30: obese). Once you do this several times, you get into the habit of organizing your data better. Always remember to name your files in a way that you can recollect what data they contain. If you cannot, make a separate file (in word, excel or notepad) listing file names and what they stand for.

3. **Background information**
I remember a review article that I wrote entitled "Current status of molecular markers for early detection of sporadic pancreatic cancer". My first attempt at writing it was in my second year of graduate school. At that time, I had not really written or published any scientific article and was just learning how to read a scientific article. I diligently collected over 500 articles, printed them off and read them. However, I realized that after about a hundred articles, there were several problems I was facing in writing the review.
a. I could not recollect what I had read in the earlier articles
b. When I went back to my notes from each article (I had written brief notes in Microsoft word), I did not have references for each note so I did not know which article to reference for a particular sentence or paragraph.

This experience taught me a valuable lesson- anticipate confusion and take steps to prevent it. So, the next time I attempted to write the article, this time in my fifth year of graduate school, I took the following steps

a. Prepared a word document which had sub headings. As I read an article, I would write a note under one of the subheadings to which the article pertained to. I would also write a few sentences before or after the central point to help explain it better and assist in maintaining flow when time came to put it all together in a single document.
b. I had software for inserting references handy (I use Reference Manager) and inserted the appropriate references soon after I wrote my summary of the article.

This time, things went much better. The end result was a twenty page review article complete with figures and tables and best of all, I felt at ease handling this mammoth of a manuscript.

## 4. Manuscript preparation
A scientific manuscript generally will comprise of the following sections
a. Title page: this contains the title, the author names, and their affiliations, keywords to identify the article in a search, and name and contact information of the corresponding author. This is best left for the end.
b. Background: This provides a brief background about why I decided to do this study. It also tells the reader succinctly what is known and what new are we trying to answer. This is one of the last sections that I write-reason being that I already know the background well enough that part of writing this section involves inserting supporting references and getting a flow in place.
c. Methods: I sometimes alternate between writing this section first with the Results section. Both of these comprise the heart of the article. The way I learnt is by reading an article written on a similar topic in a reputed journal and taking help from there to model my thoughts into words. I try to be as detailed as possible. As I am reading the finished article, I think of what I would want to know if I was a researcher trying to replicate this work. This I have found to be of immense help.

d. Results: This is the section I will usually start with. Even here, I usually organize subheadings before I start to write about the results. When I am not sure how much I should include in the write-up vs. direct them to a figure or table, I err on the side of succinctness.
e. Discussion: This is the section I plan for after I have the results. I first obtain all relevant articles, and then decide the portions of the result I want to focus on. Often I try to find articles to support or even refute our result. It makes for a healthy discussion. If you have too many references, one option would be to make a table and then write a brief summary of the tabulated results. Sometimes, a flowchart or even a diagram illustrating the overall message is very helpful. This is more common in molecular biological research where signaling pathways are depicted but can also be used in other kinds of medical research.

## 5. References

A novice to research often does not suspect that this aspect of doing research will often cause him great grief. Nowadays there are many types of software available to help with managing references including Refworks, Reference Manager and End Note. It does not matter which one you use but sticking to one is most helpful. The important thing is to get yourself familiar with how to use one of these reference management softwares before you start writing your manuscript. Most often you will use the import function to insert a reference into your manuscript. The next most common function is the "reference style" function wherein you will adjust your output to match the requirements of a particular journal. I would recommend being familiar with how to edit a given reference style to match a certain format. Many a time, you will not find the journal in the list of journals provided with the reference management software and knowing how to edit a reference style will save you time and frustrations.

## 6. Preparing to submit for peer review

Being organized while preparing your article for submission to a journal for peer review will save you lots of stress. Most common items required while submitting an article are

- A cover letter describing why your article is relevant to a given journal, introducing the authors and suggesting potential reviewers. Its best submitted on a letterhead. A sample Cover letter is included at the end of the book.
- Conflict of interest statement: This is a statement that states that you or your co authors have no vested financial interest in the work being presented.
- List of potential reviewers: These should be people who you think would be qualified to review your article. These cannot be people you have worked with or even co authors of articles with you. Sometimes these could be people you met a meeting who share similar research interests. Keeping a list of potential referees at hand will save you a lot of time.
- Copyright form: Think ahead- some journals have PDF forms that they want each author to sign and upload. So, it's important to review instructions for authors before beginning any submission process so you can get the required forms ready in advance.

# Tip 3. Plan your research in chunks

Seasoned researchers will often tell you that they have too much on their plate and are always behind their schedule. Part of the reason for that is committing too little time to too much work or underestimating the time required for a project. If you are starting out on your research career, it would be helpful to have a couple of projects on your plate- for instance, you could work primarily on data gathering for a retrospective study while at the same time doing a literature review on the same topic. Keeping two things related is easier than two distinct projects!

For residents in programs that provide the opportunity for a dedicated research time, it may be helpful to plan in advance the projects that you want accomplished during this time. One way of planning things is devote most time for the research project, lesser time for a review article and in between work on a case report (usually in the form of a poster). During busy clinical months you can work on the IRB which is generally very mundane work anyway and prepare the instruments needed for the research (e.g. learn how to use the reference and statistical software's, make a list of journals to submit your work to).

Personal issues will inevitably factor into the time you devote to research. I don't think there is any good way to get around it, so I would advice to keep your research schedule flexible. Remember, research is supposed to be enjoyable!

# Tip 4. Use whatever research time you have to do *something*, however small the task

Time is precious. We only have so much time to accomplish so many things. So, multitasking and micromanagement are key to success in research. For instance, you are in the hospital on call and you are sitting at your desk. Would you rather watch television, sleep, listen to music or complete a few more cases of that database that you are making for your retrospective study? You have the weekend off- would you spend the whole weekend relaxing or would you take some time to research on what software's are available for reference management? Even printing off a section of an article and reading it over lunch constitutes a significant component of research. Often I have sat with a blank piece of paper, a pen and my lunch and outlined my work. Ideas have an uncanny way of popping up during conversations. If not anything, go to relevant conferences. Take some time out of watching songs on YouTube to view a video on a research topic of interest. Visit websites of professional organizations like the ACP, AMA, and AGA to name a few and see what is new. Reading abstracts presented at a national meeting have often given me wonderful ideas for new research. Additionally, they also serve as a quick review of what kind of research your peers in other programs are doing.

# Tip 5. Make a start

I have a problem with starting. Be it driving, learning a new technique, or working on a new idea, I always took time to get started. I attribute part of it to fear, of failure. What if things don't go well? What will others think? But then, I tell myself, every failure is a step to success. So, once you have an idea, now is as good a time as ever to put pen to paper (or fingers to the keyboard!). Get working on that idea! In the beginning I used to review my writings every couple of minutes to count how many words I had written. It's because it was hard work. But then, it takes hard work to produce good quality work. There have been numerous times where I will start a research study, then midway find out I was doing it wrong and would have to go back and restart. It's frustrating particularly because as a resident you don't have a whole lot of time to start out with. But, when the end result comes out well it's worth it. The feeling of accomplishment is second to none. Motivate yourself however works best for you. For some small rewards or taking small steps at a time is what drives them. For others, it may be the dream of a prestigious fellowship that drives them forward. Create role models for yourself. There is nothing better than positive reinforcement!

# Tip 6. Set deadlines

For anyone familiar with the grant writing system, deadlines should come as no surprise. You have to finish your work and submit it by a certain time. Personally, I do not like deadlines in research because I feel it is something that should relax you. And in most cases of research during residency this will hold true. However, it is always good to set yourself a deadline. In this way, you will wrap up a project before you are too far out from the time of data collection. Also, from personal experience, I can say that there is a wide variation in the time between the time you first start writing an article to the time you submit it (can be from a month for a case report to a year or more for a research or review article). Once you have submitted it to a peer reviewed journal, there is an even wider variation in the time from submission to acceptance. Part of that is the factor of rejections. I once had a manuscript that was rejected a dozen times before being accepted. That being said, I also had a manuscript that was online within one month of submission. Either way, there are so many potential barriers to cross before you can have the pleasure of seeing your work in print that it is prudent to set yourself deadlines. Sometimes a key author may leave an institution before the study is submitted. This creates delays and frustrations for the others involved. Sometimes, particularly in multi-author manuscripts, it takes months to hear from everyone and then longer to achieve a consensus. One way of setting deadlines is deciding on a meeting where you want your work to be presented. Discipline in research is as important as in any other aspect of life!

# Tip 7: Work on your abstract

Abstract writing is really an art. Often, people will only read the abstract of an article. So, practice writing it. Repetition is the key. I would suggest writing separate abstracts, on different days for the same article without referring to the previous abstract. Then compare all of them. Get the abstract read by someone who is not connected to the work and see if they get enthused about your work. Read abstracts from highly cited articles and from articles in reputed journals. Then compare them with abstracts from other journals. The point here is not to belittle anyone but learn the difference in quality. Ask yourself, how much time did you spend in writing the abstract? If you were a reviewer reading your article, how would you rate the abstract? Try to make it as concise as possible without losing its meaning. Practice different kinds of abstracts- structured and unstructured. Structured abstracts will have a background, methods, results, discussion and conclusion section. Always spell-check!

As an example, I have presented two different abstracts, all in structured from for the study where we investigated the relationship between variations in liver function tests and abnormalities in red cell (anemia), white cell (leucopenia) and platelet counts (thrombocytopenia)

**Abstract 1:**

**Background:** Limited studies exist that have investigated the relationship between variation in liver function tests (LFTs) and hematologic abnormalities (anemia, leucopenia or thrombocytopenia). **Aim:** Use data from NHANES 1999-2008 to analyze the relationship between LFT levels and cytopenias. **Methods:** Demographic and laboratory data on adults 18 years and older were obtained through NHANES. Logistic regression, two point and hierarchical clustering were employed to study association between LFTs and occurrence of anemia, leucopenia or thrombocytopenia separately in males and females. **Results:** After excluding those younger than 18 years, 33560 patients remained. Forty eight percent were males. The incidence of anemia, thrombocytopenia and leucopenia in males and females was 2.8%, 0.3%, 2% and 7.7%, 0.1% and 1.9% respectively. By logistic regression, total bilirubin was the only variable significantly associated with occurrence of all three kinds of cytopenias in both genders. GGT and albumin were associated with increased odds of anemia, ALT and albumin with thrombocytopenia and albumin with leucopenia in both sexes. We identified clusters with higher relative predominance of individuals with either anemia, leucopenia or thrombocytopenia. ALT, total protein and bilirubin were the most important factors that influenced membership to one of these cluster. **Conclusion:** Variation in LFTs has significant association with occurrence of cytopenias. The relationship depends on gender and is also influenced by demographics and socioeconomic status.

## Abstract 2

**Background:** Relationship between variation in liver function tests (LFTs) (AST, ALT, Alkaline phosphatase, GGT, total bilirubin, total protein and albumin) and occurrence of cytopenias (anemia, thrombocytopenia or leucopenia) has not been well studied. **Objective:** Investigate the association between LFTs and occurrence of cytopenias in the general population by retrospective analysis of the NHANES cohort data. **Methods:** Logistic regression was employed to assess odds of developing cytopenia with variation in LFTs. Hierarchical clustering and two point analysis was used to identify groups that could be distinguished based on LFTs and cell counts. Separate analysis was carried out for males and females. **Results:** After adjusting for age, race, socioeconomic status, serum B12, folic acid, ferritin, urea nitrogen and creatinine, ALT, total bilirubin and albumin were associated with significantly lower odds of anemia. ALT was associated with decreased odds and total bilirubin with increased odds of thrombocytopenia. Total bilirubin and protein levels were associated with significantly lower and higher odds of leucopenia respectively. These associations were observed in both genders. Cluster analysis revealed groups of individuals with predominance of anemia, thrombocytopenia or leucopenia. Serum total bilirubin, age, race and poverty to income ratio were the most important variables that determined cluster membership in both genders while ALT and total protein were specifically important for males and females respectively. **Conclusion:** Significant associations exist between LFTs and occurrence of cytopenia among US adults aged 18 and older. These relationships appear to be influenced by gender and could permit identification of high risk groups for surveillance and early intervention                                                                strategies.

# Tip 8. Include informative schematics and learn the art of drawing "electronically"

It is a well known saying that a picture is worth hundreds of words. I am a very visual kind of person. So, often when going through an article, I invariably go from the abstract to its figures. A simple schematic figure sometimes goes a long way in conveying the message. An example is a checkerboard schematic showing the results of a logistic regression analysis to investigate the relationship between LFTs and cytopenias (i.e. anemia, leucopenia or thrombocytopenia).

| Male | Anemia | Thrombocytopenia | Leucopenia |
|---|---|---|---|
| AST | | | |
| ALT | | | |
| Alkaline phosphatase | | | |
| GGT | | | |
| Total protein | | | |
| Total bilirubin | | | |
| Albumin | | | |

| Female | Anemia | Thrombocytopenia | Leucopenia |
|---|---|---|---|
| AST | | | |
| ALT | | | |
| Alkaline phosphatase | | | |
| GGT | | | |
| Total protein | | | |
| Total bilirubin | | | |
| Albumin | | | |

**Figure 1.** Checkerbox schematic showing results of logistic regression analysis to investigate relationship between liver function tests and occurrence of anemia, thrombocytopenia or leucopenia. Red color indicates significantly decreased odds (i.e. odds ratio <1.0 and $p<0.05$), green color indicated significantly increased odds (i.e. odds ratio>1.0 and $p<0.05$) and grey color

indicates no significant change (i.e. p>0.05). AST (aspartate aminotransferase), ALT (alanine transferase), GGT (gamma glutamyl transferase)

From the schematic several things are apparent

- The number of significant relationships between LFTs and occurrence of cytopenias was more in females than males.
- Increased levels of ALT, total bilirubin and albumin were associated with significantly decreased odds and increasing GGT with significantly increased odds of developing anemia in males.
- All LFTs were significantly associated with occurrence of cytopenias in females.
- Total bilirubin was the only LFT associated with occurrence of all three cytopenias in both genders.

More complex diagrams can be made using a variety of software programs. I have learnt to use PowerPoint, 2007 and later versions work best for drawing complex schematic diagrams. I have found the "scribble" and "curve" tools in PowerPoint to be especially useful in drawing complex images. An example of a figure I created for one of my articles in PowerPoint can be found here http://www.ncbi.nlm.nih.gov/pmc/articles/PMC3232046/figure/F2/

# Tip 9. Choose a mentor

My first mentor was my graduate advisor. He was not just someone who advised me regarding my research but also someone I could discuss issues concerning my career and sometimes personal problems as well. My current mentor is a gastroenterologist whom I first came to know during my Ph.D. He has a strong interest in the study of pancreatic diseases and given my interest in the same, I thought he would be an ideal mentor. The other things that I also looked into while selecting my mentor were his professional interactions (I had a chance to work with him on inpatient service and found him to be very intelligent, with lots of practical knowledge and a tendency to ask questions) and publications (I researched online and on Pub Med). My final decision was based on a face to face discussion during which I found that he was someone whom I enjoyed talking to and who seemed to enjoy talking about research with me. He seemed to be genuinely interested in helping me achieve my career goals and was willing to devote some time to guiding me. Outside of these two mentors, I have had other people who have been like mentors to me. Some of them are not physicians and others are physicians with whom I am not actually doing much research but I just like discussing issues concerning professional development.

I would strongly recommend that once you have matched into a residency program, to begin looking for potential mentors. This is all the more important for those who wish to apply later on for a competitive fellowship. To answer the question "Should I have more than one mentor?" my answer would be that you should have one primary mentor who will be your go to person for most problems. Then, there should be others who would be "secondary mentors". These would be people you have interacted with, are comfortable talking to about issues, have a good rapport with you but not someone you work or discuss with on a regular basis. I also think it's a good idea to sit down early on during residency with your mentor and discuss what your goals are, where you would like his/her help, what expectations they have from you, and any suggestions for you towards planning your future career. As someone who likes to do self initiated research, I like to keep my mentor in the loop regarding manuscripts and projects sending him articles to critique. His feedback has always proven to be very valuable for me providing key clinical insight.

# Tip 10. Attend conferences

The first scientific conference I attended was a local meeting that brought together graduate students, medical students and residents to present their work. It was valuable for multiple reasons. Most importantly, it gave me an opportunity to see for myself if I had the confidence to stand in front of my poster and talk about it. I realized my biggest enemy was not fear of presentation but whether people would think my work was important enough. In the beginning, I did feel very nervous in the presence of professors and other seasoned participants but over time it has evolved into something I enjoy. The same thing for podium talks. They are more difficult because of two reasons- time constraints and interactive nature of the talk. But the advantage is that you present to a wide audience at the same time and this will improve your confidence and also get your message across.

I would suggest planning out your conferences for the year. This way you will have several advantages

- Most residency programs will want to know vacation/educational days in advance. Most have a cap on how many days residents can take off for attending conferences. By planning in advance, you can make sure conferences are not on the same months that you have clinical rotations where getting time off is either difficult or not permitted. You can also make planned use of your educational days off.

- By knowing deadlines for registration and abstract submission in advance, you can plan your research to finish before submission deadline

- For out of state conferences, prices of hotels and flights are significant concern. Knowing whether your program will fund the trip and deciding which months may be best for conferences will allow you to be economical and have an educational experience at the same time.

In my opinion there is no one conference that you should attend. Depending on what your residency is in, you may want to attend that particular societies meeting (for instance, internal medicine residents are encouraged to attend the ACP meetings). You can decide with your mentor on which conferences might be the best to attend.

# Tip 11. Take courses related to your area of interest

I was very interested in bio informatics and biostatistics. So, I took both those courses during my graduate program. That's why in residency there was no specific course that I opted for. But for those who would like to do certain types of projects (particularly those linked to epidemiology or involving biostatistics), it is helpful to search for and discus with your mentor and program leadership about enrolling early on in relevant courses. One reason that's important is because for disciplines like biostatistics, you need training in specific software programs. Often it is helpful sitting through a course for that. There are also courses available during meetings and conferences that one can attend. Further, you can also access online courses. I came across a few nice free online biostatistics courses offered by Tufts University (http://ocw.tufts.edu/Course/1/Coursehome) , Johns Hopkins (http://ocw.jhsph.edu/index.cfm/go/viewCourse/course/IntroBiostats/coursePage/schedule/) University and the University of Michigan (http://open.umich.edu/education/med/m1/patients-pop-decision-making/fall2006)

There are also some good free resources for those interested in learning how to write research papers or grants from Purdue (https://owl.english.purdue.edu/owl/section/4/16/). Some general information on academic writing can also be found at the University of Utah's website (http://ocw.usu.edu/english/intermediate-writing/index.html). I turn to Google for most of my questions. Sometimes, it takes a little sifting through but you can usually find what you need.

# Preparing your first poster- a case report

Case reports are a double edged sword. On one hand they afford us the opportunity to learn from a single case, a certain nuance of medicine. My most vivid images in medicine were those I saw in case reports. They can also act as a starting point for a search of literature, a tool to learn the analytic skills needed for larger scale research. They are also incredibly hard to publish. One portal where case reports are well received is as posters for a meeting. They provide a resident who is a novice to research, the first training at how to organize, research and present a scientific work. Unlike a manuscript, the preparation of a poster that explains a case report requires few unique tools:

- Templates: nowadays most presentations are done on PowerPoint. There are several free websites which offer templates of various sizes for download and use by the resident.
- Images: These are key to any poster particularly so for a case report. The picture of the Foley bag with purple colored urine, that rash, the virus under the electron microscope. Images are powerful and one should always strive to include images in their poster.

When you come across an interesting case, the first and foremost thing to do is to make sure you save the relevant information somewhere secure. Next, reflect on what is unique. Sometimes, I have come across cases that in isolation might not have been one of their kinds, but they taught a valuable clinical lesson. Once you have figured out the unique message that your particular patient conveys, the next thing to do is to find literature relevant to that message. For instance, let's say you had a patient present with generalized weakness. Workup revealed panhypopituitarism without any obvious cause. Serendipitously, you discovered during a routine muscle biopsy that patient has a rare form of intravascular lymphoma. In this case, the message is that intravascular lymphoma is a rare but possible cause of generalized weakness and panhypopituitarism (by clogging up the vascular supply). The next step could be looking for other reports of intravascular lymphoma in literature and investigating how many of them presented with either weakness or showed signs of hypopituitarism. Another step would be to search for potential mechanisms by which it causes various symptoms and for therapeutic trials and prognostic factors. The final step is presenting all this information together on the poster. Here again, refer, refer, refer to other posters to see how others presented their cases. Think of how you would like a poster presented if you were the visitor and finally whether your central message stands out.

Here are a list of free websites that offer poster templates for download and use

http://www.posterpresentations.com/html/free_poster_templates.html

http://www.makesigns.com/SciPosters_Templates.aspx

http://www.genigraphics.com/templates/

http://www.posters4research.com/templates.php

# Preparing your first manuscript

Writing the first manuscript is always special. My first one was a review article entitled "MUC4 as a Diagnostic Marker in Cancer" that was published in 2008. Keep the following things handy when getting ready to write a research manuscript

- Printed copies of the results. It is often easiest to write the methods and results sections first
- A printed copy of an (or more than one) article that you are going to use as a reference for style of writing.
- Using the results of your study, prepare tables and figures first. For statistical analysis, it is best to either consult previously published articles to ensure you have the right verbiage or consult a biostatistician. Also ensure you have the p-values!
- I found it very helpful to print off sections of the manuscript from time to time and review what I had written. It also helped me critically assess the writing style and make changes.
- Many journals nowadays ask for separate sections providing bulleted information on "what is already known" and "what is new". I try to include that in every article because I think those provide an important technical summary of the novelty of the study.
- After writing the first draft of the manuscript, I will print it off and read it over breaks during the day or even before bedtime. I also give it to my friends who are not directly connected with the work to see if they could get the message I was trying to convey. I have found their suggestions to be one of the most helpful.
- For residents in the early stages of their research endeavors, I would suggest that once they have a draft of their manuscript ready (with tables and figures), they should present their work in the form of a poster or oral presentation at a local or national meeting. Meanwhile the manuscript will likely make several rounds of review internally before being cleared for submission.

- More suggestions can be found in the **Be organized** section under the heading **Manuscript**
- A word of caution, save every version of the draft by a different name which can be identified later on easily. For instance MS11-16-13v1.0 means that the manuscript (abbreviated as MS) was last edited on 11-16-2013 and this is version 1.0. Subsequent versions on the same day would be 1.1, 1.2 and so on. You can use the "Compare" function under "Review" tab in Microsoft word to compare two versions of a manuscript.

# Funding

Research funding is difficult to get as a resident. However, I have found that societies representing specific residencies will often have some grants or research awards available that one can apply to. For instance, the American Medical Association has a seed grant for residents (for more information see (http://www.ama-assn.org/ama/pub/about-ama/our-people/member-groups-sections/resident-fellow-section/awards-grants.page).     Similarly, AAFP (American Academy of Family Physicians) has an award for residents (http://www.aafpfoundation.org/online/foundation/home/programs/humanitarian/familymedicinecares/fmcrsa.html).     You have to actively seek out and keep searching for resident grants. Again, I would suggest using Google and creating a word document that keeps track of grant opportunities for reference.

# Sample cover letter

Editor-in-Chief,

Life Science Journal

Dear Editor,

Please accept for your consideration for publication in the Life Science Journal the original research article entitled "Protein X as a novel marker of severity in acute pancreatitis". In this prospective single center study, we compared protein X level in serum in 50 patients with severe and 100 with mild pancreatitis. Protein X level was elevated nearly 5 fold in patients with severe pancreatitis compared to mild pancreatitis patients.

I am a resident in training in Internal Medicine at the University of Nebraska Medical center. Dr Smith is an Assistant Professor in the department of Gastroenterology and Hepatology at the Nebraska Medical center. We trust the reviewers will find this article of scientific interest for publication in your reputed journal. The undersigned author affirms that this manuscript and the data it contains are original, are not under consideration by another journal, and have not been published previously. Every author is aware of, has agreed to the content of this paper, and to being listed as an author on the paper.

If you have any questions, please contact me at (XXX) XXX XXX. Thank you for your consideration.

Looking forward to hearing from you soon.

Sincerely,

Subhankar Chakraborty,

Dept. of Internal Medicine,

University of Nebraska Medical Center. Omaha. Nebraska

# Conclusion

Every now and then we see articles in journals talking about the vanishing breed of physician scientists. The question is- how many residents have read the article? And importantly, what are the ground realities in majority of residency programs. When do residents begin their scholarly activities and to what end? How much time supposed to be dedicated to research is diverted towards clinical duties? Whatever the answers to these questions may be, research never stops. Every day, new discoveries are made. From application of existing technologies to development of novel futuristic ideas and technologies, the pace is dizzying. In this melee there is the resident physician, seeking to pursue his/her research goals. Like anything that is new, it may seem daunting in the beginning, but once you find the fun hidden inside and the joy of discovery it can be quite addictive. So, take your pen and paper (or your iPad and laptops), put your thinking caps on and begin....the world has too many questions and not enough people to answer them all....enjoy!

# About the author

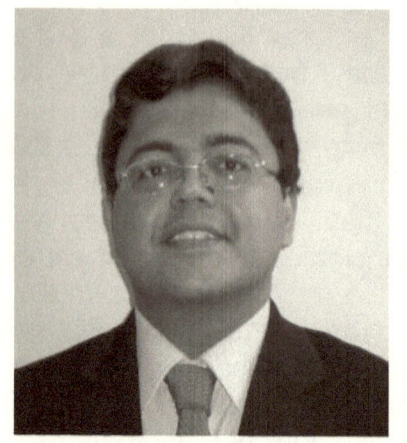

Dr Subhankar Chakraborty completed his undergraduate medical training in India from Andhra Medical College. Afterwards, he moved to the United States to do his Ph.D. in Biochemistry and Molecular Biology at the University of Nebraska medical center. Following completion of his graduate training, he started his residency in Internal Medicine at the University Of Nebraska Medical Center. He has authored or co authored nearly 50 research and review articles. He has also presented at several regional and national meetings. He is the Editor in Chief of three journals, Oncology Gastroenterology and Hepatology Reports, the International Journal of Medicine and Public Health and Free Radicals and Antioxidants. He is also part of the Editorial Board in several journals and has reviewed articles for several journals.

www.ingramcontent.com/pod-product-compliance
Lightning Source LLC
Chambersburg PA
CBHW021447170526
45164CB00001B/426